I0772489

Mindful Eating

By Jeff Cannon Copyright © 2018 by Jeff Cannon

Simple Truth LLC
1 Little West 12th Street
New York, NY 10014, info@simple-truth.com

Ordering Information:
Orders by U.S. bookstores and wholesalers please contact the publisher at the address above. Quantity special discounts are available on quantity purchases by corporations, associations, and others. For details, contact the publisher at the address above.

Printed in the United States of America
Publisher's Cataloging-in-Publication data
Cannon, Jeff.

Mindful Eating / Jeff Cannon
p. cm. ISBN: 978-1984122971

Library/Academic ISBN: 978-1466497382

1. Diet. 2. Weight Loss 3. Wellness 4. Meditation. 5. Self Help. 6. Mind and Body. 7. Personal Transformation. 8. Enlightenment I. Cannon, Jeff. II. Title.
HF0000.A0 A00 2011
299.000 00–dc22 2010999999

First Edition, January 2018
9 8 7 6 5 4 3 2

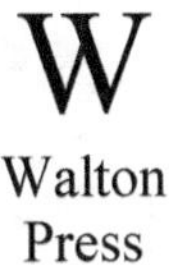

Walton
Press

**Note: The author of this work does not dispense medical advice or prescribe the use of any technique as a form of treatment for physical, emotional, or medical issues without the advice of a physician either directly or indirectly. The intent of the author is only to offer information of a general nature to help you in your search for your higher self and wellbeing.

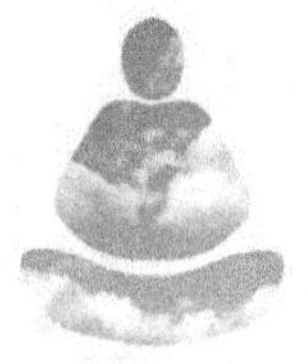

Acknowledgements

I would like to acknowledge the wonderful people I worked with on this project. My longtime designer who has always showed such skill, and artistry in everything she does, Dena Hynes, and my wonderful editor Cynthia Kling.

I would also like to thank the nutritionists and medical professionals who helped me define a healthy approach to my work.

I could not have done this without any of you.

Mindful Eating is about more than fitting into a size 2. Mindful Eating is about fitting perfectly into the body you were given no matter what size you are. It is about rising above and shedding the weight and the toxins that have held you down in body, mind, and spirit, and have prevented real you from rising above and shining through.

Part cleanse, part nutritional reset, part lifestyle modification, it is time to throw away your scale and change your mindset forever. Stop counting individual calories as you learn to cultivate new habits that will simplify your life naturally and organically as you become the person you were meant to be all along.

As you will learn, when you eliminate the toxins and excesses from your body your mind will mirror those changes in every aspect of your life.

The weight you lose in your body will be mirrored throughout every aspect of your life, mentally and spiritually, as you transform yourself without the stress of dieting and with less effort than you ever thought possible.

Eating mindfully is about enjoying the moments of awakening you never knew existed. It is about seeing the world and yourself through cleaner, sharper lenses and discovering how wonderful it is to be your own beautiful self no matter what the world throws at you.

Mindful Eating will help you remove the negative emotions and toxins that are buried deep within the weight you feel as if you are chained to. It will free you from the psychological bulk and spiritual baggage you have dragged around for far too long. It will replace the unhealthy habits from your diet and your life so that you can make the right choices you have always wanted to make without even thinking about them.

It's time to wake up and find that you can not only transform the way you eat but the way you live.

The old adage *you are what you eat* is only part of the equation today. It is not just *what* you eat it is also *how* you eat that matters. Both reflect how you feel about yourself. Stuffing yourself with whatever is available as quickly as possible so that you can get on to the next task is a reflection of your self-worth. In truth it is no different than how you dress or act, and it is time to change all of that.

Mindful Eating will gently guide you to stop rushing through your meals. You will learn to slow down and connect with the food in front of you. When you do that your food will not just nourish your body but your mind and spirit as well.

Take a moment to remember the truly exceptional meals you have had in your life. They nourished more than your body, they nourished your mind and your soul as well. They created memories that shaped you into the person you are today.

This is why it is not just enough to feed your body. You need to create a deeper and richer relationship with your meals, your food and the community around you. These are what will open the doors to a healthier relationship with yourself, a relationship that will open the door to create a community with those who truly care about you.

With your first mindful bite, you will discover a path that will only widen as you learn that eating the right food in the right way is the gateway to creating a happier, healthier, more balanced you. It will make you look and feel better no matter what body type you were born with. It will open doors to wonderful opportunities as it helps you turn your meals into experiences that will last a lifetime.

What follows is not a traditional diet. It is a lifestyle that will balance your needs with the life you want so that you can live your life, your way, and on your terms. Once you begin you will watch your body tighten and your skin clear, you will feel an awakening blossom within you as you bear witness to all of those moments of personal enlightenment that you may have never realized even existed.

Just be aware that your body's needs may differ from the guidelines within this book. That is fine, that is why they are called guidelines. Everyone is different, feel free to adjust this approach to meet the realities of your life. Most important, discuss your diet and your lifestyle with a qualified healthcare professional. Make sure your choices work with who you are. The worst thing you can do is try to be someone you're not. After all, is your life, it is up to you to decide how you want to live it.

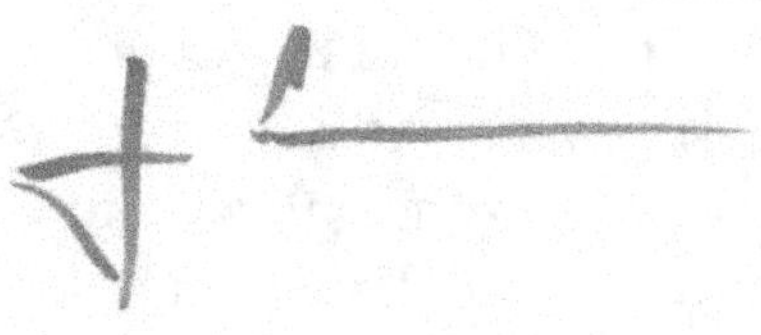

** The author of this work does not dispense medical advice or prescribe the use of any technique as a form of treatment for physical, emotional, or medical problems without the advice of a physician either directly or indirectly. The intent of the author is only to offer information of a general nature to help you in your search for greater well-being.

Every religion recognizes food as a sacrament and every meal as a sacred event. When you eat mindfully you will return to a simpler time. You will see your meals and snacks as powerful threads that connect you to the energy of life. You do not need to eat mindfully at every meal. You can take baby steps, exploring what it feels like at a lunch or a dinner to start. You can see how you feel eating mindfully several times a week. Once you get the ball rolling it will expand and grow on its own and you will be amazed at how quickly your transformation will take hold.

The more you eat mindfully the more you will notice a change in the way you think about food. You will learn to turn a simple meal into a transformative event that will take you well beyond health and weight loss. You will learn to approach life more deeply, more passionately, and more personally. The habits you create at the table will extend into the work you do, the people you know and the life you live. Every meal will become an event that nourishes your body and awakens your mind and spirit as well.

There are several ways mindful eating will help you beyond just weight loss. When you eat mindfully, you will:

- **Enjoy** your food more deeply. Research shows that taste buds lose the ability to discern subtle differences in food after eating just a small amount. Eating with greater awareness allows you to enjoy your food longer, well after the flavors have faded.
- **Slow** down your experience and give yourself time to feel satisfied with smaller portions. Studies tell us that it takes about twenty minutes to realize your stomach is full. The more time you take to eat your meal the less likely you will be to overeat.
- **Grow** more mindful of your food you gain awareness of your cravings and the difference between emotional and nutritional eating, before you reach for that cupcake or fast food burger.
- **Relieve** yourself of stress- and emotion-driven eating habits. Comfort foods may provide an emotional escape but they often result in large, carb-laden meals. Control your stress and you control your need to escape in your next meal.

From this point forward, do just one thing - stop rushing through every meal. You have time, your food is not going anywhere.

First, before every meal take a moment to sit and observe your surroundings. Take a deep, low breath down into your belly. Slow everything down. Count to six as you inhale in a nice even pace and pause your breath for a count of two before slowly releasing your breath into the room around you for another count to six. With each breath in allow yourself to settle into your seat a bit more. Give yourself permission to relax and be mindful as you acknowledge what is around you. Notice the sights, the sounds, the feelings you are experiencing. Scroll through your five senses so that you are truly present no matter where you are. Then settle into your sixth sense, that of your heat. Do not judge your surroundings, simply be aware of them.

Next, set your intention for your meal. You may simply give thanks for the food in front of you. You may wish to thank yourself for taking the time to stop and nourish your body. You may extend that thanks to your mind and spirit.

You may acknowledge that the meal before you is not the healthiest choice, but in this crazy world this is just fine until your next meal. Forgive yourself and give yourself permission to enjoy it anyway. This is a part of letting go of whatever else is going on in your life.

Once again place your awareness on the food before you. Scroll through your senses. Notice the colors before you. If it is a grey mass then acknowledge it. Do not judge it, simply remind yourself to choose something different next time; perhaps more vibrant, more colorful, perhaps something healthier. Smell the aroma of your food. Notice how your body responds as you do. Are you salivating? Are you excited? Are you disappointed? Whichever it is, use that as a reminder for whatever it is you are going to have at your next meal.

Touch. Contrary to what your parents may have said, it is okay to play with your food. snap a bean and see how it responds. Is it firm or soft? Press your fork into your mashed sweet potatoes. Are they solid or do they run with liquid? Again, do not judge your choices, simply acknowledge what it is. Be honest and aware and note your reactions. Now, take a moment to listen to your food. Does it snap, crackle or pop? Is it crisp when you cut into it? Should it be? Is it fresh or packaged? Again, do not judge, simply remember your reaction so that you will know what to order next time.

Finally, taste. Bring a bite of whatever it is you are eating to your mouth. Take a moment to let it just settle onto your tongue. Is it salty or sweet, sour or spicy? What is the texture like? Savor the flavors and the sensations of your food. Notice how your body responds to it. Are you salivating? Is your stomach rumbling? Is your throat already working?

Are you disappointed?

Be fully in your present moment and use your senses to connect with your meal.

Be fully aware of where you are and what is before you. Note the surroundings, the service and the meal you are about to enjoy, what it is doing to you and for you?

Bring your heart into your meal. Give thanks to the people who raised and farmed your food. Give thanks to the people who drove your food to your store or delivered it to your table.

Recognize that your food did not just appear in front of you but was the work of a collective of people that you should be grateful for.

Every time you enjoy a mindful meal try to transform your relationship with your food and experience the world on another level. Every bite will make you more aware of what you are putting into your body. You will also grow more aware of what it took to bring your food to you on every level. Learn to calm your senses and quiet your emotions so that for the next few minutes are not just eating a meal, you are experiencing your life free from stress, strain and tension, as you connect with those around you. Be present and in the moment while you eat but also appreciate your food fully.

When you have finished your meal, take a moment to acknowledge the food you just ate. Acknowledge the experience you just enjoyed and how it made you feel. Just as important, acknowledge that you just gave yourself time - the most precious gift any of us have these days.

You will find that in very little time your eating habits will begin to change as well as also your shopping and buying habits. You will start to look forward to your meals as a way to reduce stress and rebalance your life. You will find that it takes no more time to do this than it does to eat a meal. You may even find that shopping for your food becomes less of a chore and more of a mindful experience in itself.

A habit is not just some cloud you walk into. It is a hardwired response to the stimulus of the world around you. When you change a habit, you reprogram your brain to respond differently. It is why the way you think about food is as important as the food you eat. The habits you create with Mindful Eating will transform the way you think about life. When you transform the way your brain processes your body's needs with something as simple as food you begin to transform the way you process all kinds of information. That means as you become more aware of your food you become more aware of the media you absorb, the people you hang out with, and the world around you. Healthy choices in food create healthy choices in life.

Simplify:

Many people are confused with the diets that fill the media. Vegan or vegetarian, paleo or fusion, imported or local, fast or slow; there are so many diets that focus on the minutiae that you can fail to see the forest for the trees. No matter how your tastes run the most important part of your diet is to simplify it and return to the basics.

Your body was designed to digest unprocessed food, so that is what you need to give it. Ask yourself, is your diet basically processed or unprocessed? Is it driven by carbohydrates or proteins? I am not a dietician, but I do know eating the freshest, cleanest, food found as close to the source as possible is the best step you can take to living a healthier, happier, fitter life.

Forego the sauces, omit the extra ingredients, think instead about clean food that relies on natural spices to bring out the flavor of whatever it is you are about to enjoy.

If you find it confusing think about this. Sauces were originally created to hide the flavor and smell of rotted fish and meats. A cheese sauce on a nice piece of fish does not enhance the flavor it hides it.

Learn to let your food shine through. Learn to seek out dishes that were originally created by the hunters, gardeners and fishermen, people who had fresh ingredients on hand and not a lot of other things.

For example, paella is a simple dish originally cooked over an open fire by hunters who were far from home. Risotto is a simple way to simmer rice over an open fire transforming it into an experience within itself. Tagines, stir fries, steaming, all of these are ways of cooking that were created to make the best of the ingredients and the materials on hand. Mirror these techniques with fish, chicken, even tofu and forget about layering your food with unnecessary flavors. That is the key to quick, yet simple meals that work.

Simplify, simplify, simplify, and rely on fresh flavors not gimmicks. Let your diet transform itself naturally and it will do so for the better.

Create Your Pattern for Living

Your body is an incredible machine. It has evolved over hundreds of thousands of years. During that time your ancestors rarely ate the cleanest, healthiest food there was. They ate whatever was available, whenever it was available. Know that your body will survive the occasional indulgence. It does not care if every bite adheres to some stringent standard. What it cares about is that you are getting enough nutrients and that you are ingesting as few toxins as possible.

I know that you may not have the time to cook a meal every night. Many people cannot find affordable, fresh, local produce. Do what people have always done – eat the best food you can find and don't stress about it. When you slip, learn to smile and let it go. Just plan to make up for your slip at another meal.

Mindful Eating is not about keeping to a stringent eating schedule, it is about looking at the bigger picture. What is more important than absolute adherence to every detail of your diet is to create a *Pattern for Living*. Do not think in terms of calories and ounces or meal by meal, think ranges and month to month, think averages and trends. My weight my go up and down by a few pounds. I don't celebrate when it drops by a few pounds and I don't moan when I gain a few. As long as I am in the same range, I am happy.

It is better to enjoy life than it is to be someone else's idea of perfect. Think less about drawing a hard line in the sand based on the minutiae, think instead in of giving yourself healthy ranges to live within. Use those as guidelines and develop healthy habits that will help you stay within those ranges well into your future.

Always strive to eat the best food you can, but do not ruin your life for it. Understand that you will slip sooner or later, give yourself permission to slide and then let it go. Transforming your diet and your life does not happen overnight. It takes time. Stop beating yourself up because you ate 10 more calories than you should have. Focus on shifting your diet in the right direction with balanced meals based on nutritional value and the lack of additives. Enjoy what you have because far too many don't have enough.

When you listen to your body and what it is asking for, you begin to learn how your body and mind work together. When you focus on clean, simple foods and flavors, that idea will echo into every corner of your life. As the distractions fade from your plate they will fade from your life and allow your spirit to soar.

Don't Stop Eating

It may sound crazy, but if you want to find a healthy weight that you can live with, then you need to eat. When you eat you give your body the energy it needs to keep working. When your body keeps working, you keep burning calories. If you stop eating, your body slows down and you stop burning calories. A healthy diet does not mean starving yourself, but eating the right things in the right way.

The secret is to eat based on your body's needs not the needs of your mind. Keep to three healthy meals every day. Make sure they are smaller and more balanced with healthy snacks in between. Almonds, toasted and unsalted, are a perfect snack to keep your body going. Celery and almond butter is another. You can even try a slice of apple with a touch of almond butter. Are you seeing a pattern yet? It is important that you don't skip meals or replace them with sugary snacks, but that you augment your meals with healthy snacks.

Breakfast: If you skip breakfast as many do, you skip the one meal that will start your engine and keep it running for the day ahead. The calories and time you save skipping breakfast quickly leads to a lack of energy that will hit you mid-morning and result in added calories you end up eating to hold you over until lunch. Take a few minutes to eat a real breakfast[i], not a doughnut or a high-fructose fruit shake, but a slice of toast and two egg whites, or enjoy a small bowl of granola or oatmeal.

These will keep you energized, and the calories you save from not snacking will easily make up for the food on your plate.

Lunch: This should be the largest meal of your day. What you eat for lunch will keep you going well into the evening. Just make sure you have a large salad for lunch or with lunch. Combine fish or chicken to incorporate protein. Turn this into a mindful meal. Just don't feel like you have to have the double burger with fries and a shake to stock up. Think simple instead.

Dinner: Eat earlier and go lighter with your dinner. Think in terms of bed. Especially avoid carbohydrates as they will sit all night, transforming into fats for the morning. You should be winding down your day and your digestion rather than stuffing yourself with comfort food. Most important, take your time and relax, but not in front of the television as you eat.

Animals were not meant to be raised and slaughtered in a factory farm. Neither were we. There are really no natural foods that are outright bad for you; as long as they are <u>eaten in moderation</u>. We were not meant to live in a world of concrete, megabyte downloads, and 12-hour work days. The stress of their situations, and ours, is just too taxing on all of our bodies, minds and spirits.

Red meat, while not the healthiest choice, is not necessarily bad for you when eaten in small amounts and with enough time in between so that your body can properly digest it. The same is true for wine and spirits. Just make sure that whatever you eat and drink is raised and processed as naturally as possible.

Do No Harm: Non-GMO, free-range, and as humanely raised as possibly is the only approach to take. It is what you would want in your life, why continue that thread in the life of the food you consume?

Avoid Packaging: Try to avoid pre-packaged fish, meats and poultry. Opt for something you can see in a butcher's or fish-monger's case. It will be healthier for you and it will put you in closer touch with the cycle of life and death we all depend on.

Moderation: A glass of wine is not a bad thing on its own. However, if you drink a bottle every day, life can become miserable and even toxic. The same is true throughout the rest of your life. Start with the food you eat and that same concept will flow into the rest of your life.

Your body can process a lot of different kinds of foods, but this takes time. Give it the time it needs to properly digest whatever you are putting into your body. The same is true for news and information Vegetables it can digest quickly. Fish and chicken may take a day or two. Red meat and alcohol can take even longer, especially when meats are combined with starches that can leave you with unprocessed food in your gut.

As in life, success in maintaining a mindful diet is found in moderation. As you become aware of the foods you eat you will learn how they make you feel physically and emotionally. Use that as a guide to determine how often to eat any ingredient on your plate. Use this same approach to the news you watch and the social media you interact with.

The next time you order, don't rush. Pause and take a moment. Breathe slowly, find your balance, and ask yourself what you really want. Ask yourself why you are ordering what you are ordering. You will probably find that, at first, many of the things you think you want, you are actually ordering out of habit or because you ordered them the last time.

They may be easy foods that you are comfortable with. Perhaps you are tired and just want something that is quick. Whatever the reason, be mindful of the "why" behind the "what" in your diet. And yes, the same goes for the websites you visit, the news you watch and the life you live. Only you know the reasons behind why are you are eating what you eat. If you want to explore these ideas, you have to take the time to actually taste your food and learn what foods work for you and which ones don't.

At first, you may find that this is not as easy as it sounds. In time your outlook on life will change. You will stop looking at your food as a bland something you put in your mouth and chew. It will become a part of you. It will take on a new place in your life and become a source of nourishment at every level.

Start by asking yourself what is it that you really want to eat? Move past the immediate urge that you feel. Think beyond that physical craving. Think about what type of food your body is asking for?

Spend a few moments thinking about what you want in the moments before ordering. Then ask yourself how much you really need to satisfy yourself. Do you really need the extra sides? Do you really need the larger portion? You may find that you don't really want all of that – it is just your first response to seeing the bounty of food before you.

At the end of your meal, ask yourself if you feel sated, bloated, satisfied, or stuffed? You should feel clean and satisfied, but never stuffed. You should always feel as if you could enjoy a nice walk after your meal, because that is what you should always do, enjoy a nice walk.

As always, you should never judge or shame yourself when you are done with your meal, simply use how you feel as a framework for your next meal.

Judging yourself or feeling guilty is a waste of time. Just remember how you feel after you eat so that you can decide what to have at your next meal and for the choices that lay ahead for you in dining and in life. After all, it is your life to live as you want. Just be mindful so that you are truly living it your way.

Your body is a beautiful machine. Like all machines, sooner or later it comes down to numbers. By numbers, I don't mean counting individual ounces or calories, I mean general ranges and trends. Your body needs fuel in order to run. What it does not burn through exercise and simply staying alive, it stores. If you eat more than you burn, your body stores the excess as fat and you gain weight. If you burn more than you consume, then your body tires or it begins to burn its fat reserves for the energy you are missing.

This is basic math. If you eat fewer calories than you burn, you lose weight. If you eat more, you gain weight. Now that you know that, let it go.
What is left out of that equation is time. If you are n not in a hurry and would rather have a healthy approach to weight loss or weight gain, then take your time.

Keep the concept in mind, but do not obsess on the numbers. If you spend all your time counting calories one by one, your life becomes one of accounting, not living. If you are in a hurry for some event, then you should have planned ahead and given yourself more time to lose whatever weight you want to lose.

Aside from Intermittent Caloric Reductions, what is more important than individual calories, is focusing on the quality of food that you eat. Quality over quantity will help you maintain you overall health and wellness every time, and that is what we are going for here.

If you want to lose weight, replace carbohydrates with protein and replace meats with plant -based proteins. Just do so in a healthy manner. Maintain a balance that fits your lifestyle. If you eat junk, your body turns to junk. If you eat healthy, your body stays healthy. Your skin and hair and teeth and eyes will do the same, so will the people around you who are touched by your energy.

For example, a woman in the thirty to fifty age range who is moderately active burns 2,400 to 2,800 calories on average each day. A moderately active man in that same age range burns 2,800 to 3,400.

Just remember, you are different from everyone else. Some people have higher metabolic rates and burn more calories doing absolutely nothing. They can eat all day and never gain an ounce. Others can eat almost nothing and seem to retain everything. Spend less time counting and more time being. Get comfortable with who you are no matter what you see in the mirror. As for the media, and society in general, turn them off for a while.

Find your own balance, one that matches your lifestyle. Beauty is not about size but about being comfortable with your body and use that to enjoy the life you want to live.

I am not a big fan of fasting. With everything we know about the body and how it processes food, there is little reason to fast. However, I do believe in *Intermittent Caloric Restrictions*. Fasting is when you eat nothing. You become lethargic and is just not a sustainable course of action. Caloric Restrictions are when you lower your caloric intake to a low enough level that your body thinks you are entering into a time where there is no food, even though, in the modern world there is.

Losing weight is important, and you will, but it should not be the only reason you are here. Cleaning out and opening up is. This is about reducing your caloric intake to a level that maintains your metabolism while increasing your awareness of what you actually put into your body and how the toxins you put in, weight you down.

It will provide you with enough calories to maintain an active life so that you can change your old habits and transform your life in the right direction. For those who want to lose weight and keep it off, I recommend one day of caloric restriction each week. For those who want a period of mental clarity, to improve focus and remove distractions, then one day every month will certainly help.

Monitor what works for you and check with your doctor or healthcare professional so that you practice this in a safe way. When you cut back on your caloric intake you will start to realize how little food you actually need to keep you going. You will also become more aware of your cravings you used to have and of how you used to satisfy them.

As you become more comfortable with this process your day of caloric reduction will become less about food and more about the feelings of clarity and lightness that you will experience. It's simple and easy, and recognized by more and more health professionals as a healthy way to manage your weight and your life.

I started with the idea of a weekly fast and lost a lot of weight. I realized that when I ate mindfully I could do with a monthly caloric restriction instead. A key component to caloric restriction is the time you allot to it. I have found cutting my daily intake to between 600 and 800 calories one day a week is enough. By most accounts this is true for most active adults. However, check with your healthcare provider to ensure it is a healthy choice for you.

When you eat a meal, your body spends a few hours processing your food. It burns what it needs immediately and stores the rest as fat. When you restrict your calories, your body doesn't have as much energy readily available. It begins to access your stored fat and produce lean muscle mass as your body prepares itself for lean times ahead.

This will give you a leaner, healthier look and outlook with which to approach life. It is important that you not view this day of caloric restriction as a "diet." It is a day to enjoy your life. It is not enough to simply not eating. It is a day of clarity that will lead you to healthier choices before, during and after your day of caloric restrictions.

Because every calorie will count on that day, you will want to plan ahead and be even more mindful of what you eat. Because every calorie counts you will want to minimize the carbohydrates in your diet – food such as candy bars, pastries, and pasta should be avoided. You will also want to replace your regular fats with healthier fats from coconut oil, olive oil, olives, butter, eggs, avocados, and nuts

As you get used to your periodic restrictions your cravings for unhealthy food will diminish and your need for clean, healthy, beneficial foods will increase. Your body will naturally shift away from fast-burning carbohydrates to protein and healthy fats. It will also become cleaner, leaner, and tighter with fewer toxins so that you feel better.

In addition to helping you maintain a healthy weight and waistline, research has shown that fasting triggered a 1,300 percent rise of human growth hormone (HGH) in women, and an astounding 2,000 percent in men. HGH, or human growth hormone plays an important role in maintaining health, fitness and longevity by promoting muscle growth, and fat loss through increased metabolism.

In studies, caloric restriction enhanced overall health through:

- Improved biomarkers of disease
- Normalized ghrelin levels, this hormone is also known as "the hunger hormone." It is lower in obese people, and by normalizing it you remove many of the urges to eat.
- Reduced inflammation and decreasing free radical damage
- Lower triglyceride levels
- Improved memory functions and learning

According to Dr. Stephen Freedland, a professor at the Duke University Medical Center, "undernutrition without malnutrition" is an experimental approach that consistently improves survival in animals with cancer, as well as extends lifespan overall by as much as 30 percent.

Mark Mattson, a senior investigator for the National Institute on Aging, researched the health benefits of caloric restriction. His study showed that overweight adults with moderate asthma lost eight percent of their body weight after cutting their caloric intake by 80 percent every other day over for an eight-week period. In addition to that, markers for stress and inflammation decreased, and as their symptoms improved.

Mattson also researched the protective benefits of fasting and caloric restrictions to the nervous system. He states, "If you don't eat for ten to sixteen hours, your body will go to its fat stores for energy, and fatty acids called ketones will be released into the bloodstream. This has been shown to protect memory and learning functionality, as well as slow disease processes in the brain."

In the Los Angeles Times, Mr. Mattson said "In normal healthy subjects, moderate fasting — maybe one day a week or cutting back on calories a couple of days a week — will have health benefits for most anybody."

A number of other studies show that intermittent fasting and caloric restrictions can improve cognitive functions and protect against some of the damaging effects of Alzheimer's and Parkinson's diseases. According to an article in the American Journal of Clinical Nutrition the benefits may include "a decrease in blood pressure, reduced oxidative damage to lipids, protein and DNA, and an improved insulin sensitivity and glucose uptake, as well as a decrease in fat mass (Translation: You will look and feel better than ever before).

Enjoying a day of caloric restriction means eating <u>enough calories</u> to live in a normal, healthy manner. However, to start, it may mean cutting back on exercise on your day of restriction and scheduling around events that you want to attend. It may mean having two boiled eggs for breakfast and a large salad for lunch, as well as a piece of fish or chicken for dinner. It may mean eating a small handful of almonds from time to time. These are all habits that will carry over to the rest of your week.

Vegetables will become your salvation, and low-fat rather than no-fat will save you. Generally speaking, foods that are high in protein with a low glycemic index like sweet potatoes, broccoli, cauliflower, eggplants, natural muesli, natural oats, cherries, apples and plums are what you want.

Drink lots of water and stay hydrated. Also, when you feel hungry, try to wait ten to fifteen minutes before you eat to see if your hunger subsides. Your goal is to have food that makes you feel satisfied, but stays within your caloric range.

Here are two sample meals to get you started. They illustrate what an approximately 600 – 800 calorie day looks like. These guidelines will give you an idea of what it takes to enjoy a day of restriction. Adjust it to your needs, change each to fit your preferences. As with everything with Mindful Eating adapt to make them your own needs.

600+ Calorie Day
Breakfast: Enjoy a light, fast, protein rich start:

Coffee or tea w/almond milk	5
Boiled egg [egg white only]	34
Small arugula salad [handful]	3

Lunch: **Bulk up with low-calorie greens:**

Spinach salad:	300

8 c. spinach, ½ grilled chicken breast
½ c carrots, cucumber, tomatoes, etc.

Snack: **Hold your hunger with a simple snack:**

½ Banana	55

Dinner: **Think of it, you just have a few hours to go:**

Salmon filet [6 oz]	190
Small salad [6 oz]	30
Total:	617

800+ Calorie Day

Breakfast: Light, fast, & protein rich:

Coffee w/almond milk	5
2 boiled eggs [yolks removed]	34
Small arugula salad [handful]	3

Lunch: Bulk up with low-calorie greens:

Spinach salad	372
8 c. spinach, 1 grilled chicken breast	
½ c. carrots, cucumber, tomatoes	

Snack: Hold hunger with a simple snack:

¼ Cup almonds	206

Dinner: Almost There:

Salmon filet [6 oz]	190
Small salad [6 oz]	30
Total:	840

You will notice is that it does not take a lot to jump from 600 to 800 calories. Pace yourself and plan in advance so that you can reap the benefits of healthy calorie reduction.

What you eat is up to you. You have control over the dietary decisions that you make every day. In fact, you have control over all the decisions that you have to make at any point in time. If you teach yourself to stop, to breathe and to think before making those decisions you can steer your life in the direction you want it to go. Why not start with the food you eat? When you do you will train yourself to make all of your decisions in a more mindful manner throughout your life.

Instead of simply rushing into your next meal, stop, breathe and think about what you really want. Take a moment to ask yourself why you are eating what you are eating. Is it from an emotional urge? It is from habit? Or is it because that is what you truly feel like eating?

Whatever it is, here are some guidelines to follow. They will help you clean up your diet. They will also teach your brain a new way to process the other decisions you make without even thinking about it They will also provide some foods to avoid to start making good choices in your diet and in your life.

The Trouble with Sugar
So many nutritionists talk about cutting sugar from your diet it almost seems redundant to mention it here, but it is such an important part of creating a more balanced and nutritious lifestyle that I am compelled to do so. If you remember one thing it should be this, **sugar = fat**.

The trouble with sugar started thousands and thousands of years ago. Your body was created for survival. Back then storing excess energy was a key part of that. When food was abundant your body stored whatever was not immediately used in the form of fat. In lean times, when food was scarce, your ancestors survived on those reserves of stored fat. In today's world of processed foods and high fructose sweeteners, this ancient survival technique has become a death sentence for many people.

The problem is, your body doesn't know it is living in the contemporary world of the 21st century. Your body still sees sugar as instant energy. It is fast burning and short lasting. What you don't use right away can be stored as fat at a later time.

When you eat sugar the level of glucose in your blood stream rises. This stimulates the pancreas to release insulin. The release of insulin makes it difficult for your body to convert the sugar into a form that can be used right away and your body stores what remains as fat. And your body has an uncanny ability to store a lot of fat.

As if this weren't enough, sugar also happens to be the basic building block of carbohydrates. When you eat a carbohydrate (i.e., bread, pasta, candy, beer, wine) you are basically eating sugar. When your body breaks the carbohydrates down the resulting sugar is all that is left. Once again, that sugar raises the level of glucose in your blood stream, releasing insulin and starting the cycle all over. If you can't remember that, keep this in mind: you can't process that sugar unless you are very, very active.

You crave sugar and carbs because your body thinks they are survival food. But your body was not created for a world with a fast food chain on every corner. The sugars that used to keep you alive burn so fast that they fail to give you the nutrients you need, especially with today's processing and refining techniques.

When you eat them, you get a quick burst of energy followed by a crash. It is why sugar-loaded snacks pick you up and then leave you feeling lethargic, irritable, and hungry again. Your response is to grab another sugary snack which sends you on another rollercoaster of sugar highs and hunger crashes that spiral you downward.

Marketers know this, which is why the starchy, sugary treats are all that fill the shelves of every convenience store free of any antioxidants, vitamins, minerals or fiber that your body needs to sustain itself and you in a healthy manner. Hence the term, empty calories – you get calories from the sugar without the nutrients your body needs for the long haul. This is why sugar is one of the most misunderstood food groups there is. Your body loves the taste but they lack the sustenance that you need to survive.

When you cut the sugars out of your diet you cut out a tremendous problem in your health - physically, mentally and spiritually. When you replace carbohydrates with protein, and empty calories with whole grains and vegetables, you shift your entire thinking. You stop searching for quick fixes and start pursuing healthy choices. When you choose proteins over carbohydrates you begin to balance your diet for a leaner, lighter, happier life based on healthy decisions.

That craving you have for pizza or wine? The urge you have for a cupcake? That is your body saying it wants more sugar. When you give into that craving, you start the old cycle and give into your primordial self. When you overcome your addiction to sugar, and it is a physical addiction, you will change the way you think. Instead of running after the next shiny distraction, like a candy bar, you will start to look for real nutrition that will keep you going for the long term; and yes, that will extend to how you live your life, including the friends you follow, the career you pursue, and the entertainment you chase after.

Just be careful that you do not cut carbohydrates out of your diet all together. You need some healthy carbohydrates to stay well. Healthy carbohydrates help your liver produce glycogen. Glycogen safeguards your body against dehydration and muscle loss. If you stop eating carbohydrates completely your liver will stop producing glycogen and your risk of dehydration and muscle loss can increase. This is why people who exercise a lot can eat healthy carbohydrates. Their bodies burn fast, so they need those carbohydrates to fuel their fires.

Doctors suggest that you should consume at least 100 grams of healthy carbohydrates every day. These can come from vegetables, cheese, lentils or black beans, as well as fruits or nuts.

The choice is yours – healthy carbs that keep your metabolism up and your body running smoothly, or empty carbs that quickly run you into the ground and leave you with nothing but a spare tire.

Your body evolved eating rough and raw food. When sugar, rice or flour is refined, all the natural bran, vitamins and minerals are stripped away. What is left is a simple carbohydrate and your body has a problem digesting simple carbohydrates. They lack the proteins, vitamins and minerals that your body needs to properly digest, or metabolize these carbohydrates. Without those essentials your body only partially metabolizes the carbohydrates and the creation of a toxic metabolite can result.[vi]

These metabolites can interfere with the normal respiration of your cells. Yes, your cells breathe. When they don't get enough oxygen to function normally, they die. This is why refined sugar has been called "lethal" by many doctors. Because sugar only provides empty calories, your body actually leaches the necessary vitamins and minerals from your bones and organs to replace the ones that were stripped out during the refining process.

If you want to eat bread – make sure it is whole wheat, oat or seven-grain. Do the same with unpolished brown rice. Nature provides you with food that will keep your body in balance. The further you wander from the natural state you go, the worse the food is for you. As a general rule, stay away from white food. Look for food with the natural minerals and vitamins in place. They are there for a reason.

Alcohol is Sugar

The human body was not designed to digest alcohol. It is basically a toxin. But so are the cities you live in, the stress you feel, and the 24/7 lifestyle you find yourself in. Your body was not designed for any of this, so while drinking alcohol is not recommended, if you want to enjoy a sip every now and then, do so, but do so in moderation.

From a dietary point of view, beer, wine, scotch or vodka are carbs because they turn into sugar. It is a primary reason for a hangover. It is also a primary reason why alcohol quickly leads feeling and looking bloated.

Avoid alcohol if you can. If not, enjoy it in moderation. Enjoy it with the idea of quality over quantity. If you want to lose weight, avoid it all together. If your lifestyle leads you to have a sip or two, then make a conscious decision to give yourself a cutoff before you start.

Apply the idea of Mindful Eating when you drink. Do not just gulp down as much as you can, take the time to smell, to taste, to enjoy the euphoria it brings. Enjoy the stress it removes, even if only for a moment.

If you do want a drink every now and then, just know that wine is one of the worst sugar offenders. Brown alcohols like scotch comes next. The impurities that provide their color and flavor also provide a lot of toxins. Whatever you decide upon, enjoy it in moderation and think before you sip.

More Fiber

If you want to live a healthier life and create a healthier diet then you need to eat more fiber. Few people eat enough fiber, and I can almost guarantee that thanks to refined and processed foods, you are not eating enough of it.

Good dietary fiber is important to your health because it cleans and balances your system It helps your meal last longer so that you feel full and satisfied longer. It also helps to normalize your digestive system and helps to control your cholesterol and manage your blood sugar levels.

High fiber diets are what dieticians call "energy dense." That is, they have fewer calories for the same volume of food eaten. Good dietary fiber is found in fruits, vegetables, whole grains and legumes.

How much fiber do you need? The institute of medicine says a man aged 51 or older needs about 38 grams a day. A woman of the same age needs 21 grams. As a reference, 24 almonds is roughly 3.3 grams of fiber, a cup of cooked white rice is about 1.4 grams, and a cup of cooked brown rice is 3.5 grams of fiber. As with calories, you do not need to count every bit of fiber you eat. Instead, get a general feel for what your needs are and adjust.

A good way to approach fiber is to simply start eating a salad or some greens at every meal. Teach yourself to stop eating a sandwich for lunch and start eating a salad. Add tofu or vegetarian dishes instead of steak or chicken if you wish.

According to a 2012 study by the Institute of Medicine, the average man, 51 years or older generally requires 30 grams of fiber daily. The average woman of the same age generally requires 21 grams daily.

As with calories, you do not need to count grams of fiber every day. Use them as guidelines and just remember to add more vegetables to your meals.

As you clean the toxins from your system you may start to become aware of sensitivities to different foods. You may notice that some foods like yeast increase your sensitivity to pollen and other allergens. Other food, like dairy products, may cause you to become congested or to feel gassy or bloated. These are not food allergies – they are mild reactions that you simply have not noticed before. They usually do not lead to the kind of deadly reaction that some people have to nuts, but they can cause discomfort. Such food sensitivities do not mean you cannot eat cheese or wheat or yogurt at all, they simply mean that you need to find the right balance that works for your body.

There are no hard lines to food sensitivities because it is all about your saturation point. Yu need to find the level at which your body can tolerate what you are eating. You need to moderate your consumption to where you can safely eat something rather than cutting it out all-together. Before you start testing the foods you eat, check with a qualified medical professional to ensure you are aware of any allergies you may have. If you are allergic to a certain food, do not attempt to modify your diet –

Do not eat it at all.

For those foods that cause mild discomfort to your lifestyle, think about taking a two-step approach to transforming your diet. First, train yourself to be aware of how you feel after you eat different foods. Some key ingredients to watch for are dairy products, red meat, grains and breads. Take note of how you feel after you have eaten them.

For those foods that you can connect to a physical or emotional change, you may want to test them yourself. **Initiation** is the time for you to cut back on those foods. Remove them from your diet for ten days. It may be tough. Your cravings for them may increase. You may have the urge to binge. But if you can cut them out for ten days, you have taken a tremendous leap in overcoming your body's physical addiction to them. You might notice a difference in how you feel, even how you act. You may find that you are calmer or that your digestion has become more balanced. You may find that some of your cravings are gone.

Replacement. In replacement you can begin to introduce some of the foods you removed during Induction. This does not mean you can now run out and gorge on sweets or breads or cheese. It means you can reintroduce them into your diet in small amounts. See if your reactions come back. If so, you need to think about moderating how much you eat or even find a replacement for it.

If you react badly to milk, you may try soy or almond milk. If cheese makes you bloated you may decide to cut it out of your diet except for an occasional dinner. The key is not to simply return to where you were before, but to be mindful of the foods you want to reintroduce into your diet. Set limits for different foods or omit them all together.

Again, it all depends on you as an individual and what is a healthy balance for your body.

There are very few good things about processed food other than the fact that it has longer shelf-life. If you are committed to living a healthier life cut out as much processed food as possible. The reason is simple: the more a raw food is processed the fewer *real* calories it has. Pound for pound, processed meats and chips have less real nutrition compared to the levels of sugar, salt and additives they carry.

That means your body is packing away more pounds and getting less fuel with every bite. Your body is also being filled up with additives that can do more harm than good. From genetically modified seeds to corn syrup, monosodium glutamate, artificial sweeteners, Nitrates and Nitrites, your body is ingesting ingredients which maintain shelf life but do nothing else. While some food additives are worse than others, here is a list of what I consider the worst offenders. Use is as a first step toward living a healthier, happier, longer life.[viii]

Artificial Sweeteners

Aspartame is found in all types of diet or sugar free foods. It is more commonly known through such brand names that I cannot mention here. It is believed to be carcinogenic and has a range of adverse reactions associated to it. In fact, some say it has more adverse claims than all other foods and food additives combined. Aspartame is known as a neurotoxin and is said to affect short-term memory and intelligence. The components of this toxic sweetener may lead to a wide variety of ailments including brain tumors, lymphoma, diabetes, Alzheimer's, fibromyalgia, and chronic fatigue as well as depression and anxiety, dizziness, headaches, nausea, migraines and seizures. Aspartame can be found in diet sodas, jello and gelatins, desserts, gum, drink mixes, baking goods, table top sweeteners, cereal, mints, puddings, ice tea, as well as chewable vitamins and toothpaste.

High Fructose Corn Syrup

High fructose corn syrup (HFCS) is a highly-refined artificial sweetener. It has become the number one source of calories for Americans. It is found in almost all processed foods. HFCS increases weight faster than any other ingredient. It increases your LDL (bad cholesterol levels), and contributes to the development of diabetes and tissue damage, among other harmful effects. HFCS can be found in most processed foods, breads, candy, flavored yogurts, salad dressings, canned vegetables, and cereals

Monosodium Glutamate (MSG)

MSG is an amino acid used as a flavor enhancer in soups, salad dressings, chips, frozen entrees, and many restaurant foods. MSG is known as an excitotoxin, a substance which overexcites cells to the point of damage. Studies show that regular consumption of MSG may result in adverse side effects which include depression, disorientation, fatigue, headaches, and obesity. MSG affects the neurological pathways of the brain and disengages the "I'm full" function which explains some effects of weight gain. MSG can be found in prepared food, snacks, chips, cookies, seasonings, frozen dinners, lunch meats

Trans Fat

Trans fat is used to enhance and extend the shelf life of food. Many think it is one of the more dangerous substances you can consume. It is found in deep-fried and processed foods made with margarine or partially hydrogenated vegetable oils. Trans fats are formed through hydrogenation and studies show that trans fat increases LDL cholesterol levels while decreasing HDL ("good") cholesterol. It increases the risk of heart attacks, heart disease and strokes, and contributes to increased inflammation, diabetes and other health problems. Trans fats can be found in: margarines, chips, crackers, baked goods, fast foods

Food Dyes

Studies show that artificial colorings that are found in soda, fruit juices and salad dressings may contribute to behavioral problems in children and lead to a reduction in IQ. Animal studies have linked some food colorings to cancer. While not all bad, some to avoid include:

- **Blue #1 and Blue #2**
  Banned in Norway, Finland and France. May cause chromosomal damage. Found in some candy, cereal, soft drinks and sports drinks.

- **Red dye # 3 Red #40**
  Banned in 1990 after 8 years of debate, this dye has been proven to cause thyroid cancer and chromosomal damage in laboratory animals. It is still being used today and may also interfere with nerve transmission in the brain. It can be found in fruit cocktails, maraschino cherries, cherry pie mix, ice cream, and candy.

- **Yellow #6 and Yellow Tartrazine**
  Banned in Norway and Sweden this may increase kidney and adrenal gland tumors in laboratory animals. It may also cause chromosomal damage. Yellow #6 can be found in: American cheese, macaroni and cheese, candy and carbonated beverages.

6. Sodium Sulfite (E221)

Preservative used in wine-making and other processed foods, according to the FDA asthma and sulfites. Individuals who are sulfite sensitive may experience headaches, approximately one in 100 people is sensitive to sulfites. There is a suggested link between breathing problems and rashes. Sodium Sulfite can be found in wine and dried fruit.

Sodium Nitrate/Sodium Nitrite

Sodium nitrate and sodium nitrite are preservatives, as well as colorings and flavorings. These ingredients have been found to be highly carcinogenic. It forms a variety of compounds that can affect internal organs including the liver and pancreas. The USDA tried to ban these additives in the 1970's but was vetoed. Nitrates and Nitrites can be found in: hotdogs, bacon, ham, luncheon meat, cured meats, corned beef, smoked fish and many other processed meats.

BHA and BHT (E320)

Butylated hydroxyanisole (BHA) and butylated hydrozyttoluene (BHT) are common preservatives that keep foods from changing color or becoming rancid. It effects the brain's neurological system, alters behavior and has cancer causing potential. They are found in potato chips, gum, cereal, frozen sausages, enriched rice, lard, shortening, candy.

Sulfur additives are toxic. In the United States of America, the FDA has prohibited their use on raw fruit and vegetables. Adverse reactions include: bronchial, hypotension (low blood pressure), flushing tingling sensations or anaphylactic shock. It also destroys vitamins B1 and E. The International Labor Organization says to avoid E220 if you suffer from conjunctivitis, bronchitis, emphysema, bronchial asthma, or cardiovascular disease. Sulfur Dioxide is found in beer, soft drinks, dried fruit, juices, cordials, wine, and potato products.

Potassium Bromate

An additive used to increase volume in some white flour, breads, rolls; potassium bromate is known to cause cancer in animals.

SUMMARY

Now that you have learned some of the concepts behind Mindful Eating, it is time to refine your own Mindful Diet in a way that works for you. What follows is a general outline to creating a healthier, happier, more aware relationship with your food. Just remember it is important to understand that you are different from everyone else. Your body, your metabolism, your individual needs are your own. Take the time to check with a certified healthcare professional to ensure these recommendations will work for you.

Take the time to be mindful when you eat. It starts when you decide what you want to eat, when you shop or when you order your food. Teach yourself to stop, breathe and think before you act.

Simplify your food. Increase the roughage and fiber in your diet, it helps balance your system and will help you to stay full longer.

Remove processed carbohydrates from your diet and try to consume natural carbohydrates every day. These can come from vegetables, cheese, lentils, black beans as well as fruits or nuts.

Remove white flour, white sugar and white rice from your diet. Switch to their more natural states like whole grain breads. Use brown rice or switch to natural grains such as quinoa or wild rice.

Remove all doughnuts, cookies, cupcakes and fancy pastries from your diet. They are the empty calories to avoid.

Remove artificial sweeteners. Use honey, or natural cane or beet sugar if you need a sweet fix, the body can process them in moderate amounts.

Remove all processed foods. The more a food has been touched by machines the worse it becomes for you. No lunch meats, no chips, no sodas, no refined pastries or desserts. Eat foods as close to their natural state as possible. They have shorter shelf lives but create longer human lives

Think Caloric Restriction. One to two days a week reduce your caloric intake to approximately 600 – 800 calories depending on your needs. Remember, 1 pound of fat equals approximately 3,500 calories.

Review the foods that you eat and the reactions you have to them. Identify which foods lead to an adverse reaction. Create an informal Induction and Replacement program for yourself and assess each food based on the severity of your reaction, as well as the level of pleasure it brings you.

Live Your Life. No diet is worth undermining your ability to enjoy the life you are living. So temper whatever you decide to do with the understanding that you were put here for a reason. Enjoy the life that you have. But do it with moderation and in a mindful way. You don't have to look like anyone else. You don't have to be a size 2 model. You simply need to be comfortable with who you are in a healthy way. That is the true secret to being beautiful.

You will slip, you will stumble. Do not worry, simply expect it. Do not judge yourself or shame yourself. Simply use each slip as a lesson and let it go. When you get the urge for something, pause, take three deep breaths and ask yourself what it is that you really want? Teach yourself to stop rushing after your urges and think instead of what would be good for you. You have spent a lifetime creating habits and addictions for yourself. They will not disappear overnight. When you realize how food can be a replacement for your emotional needs, you will realize why it is important to manage your food and not let it manage you.

Begin today and take baby steps toward a new you and you will learn how quickly your life will fall into order. I will always be here for guidance.

WEEK1-2: Limit Your Carbs

Start small and take baby steps. It's the best way to ensure success as you explore your new life and walk down your path to uncover the beauty that has always been within.

Make a habit of breathing mindfully before, during and after your meals. Connect to your food and to the people around you and the space around you. Give thanks for the food before you and enjoy a greater connection to your food.

Remove the following foods from your diet:
- Foods made with sugar or corn syrup.
- White flour, white sugar, white rice
- Alcohol

WEEK 3 – 4 [day of caloric restriction]
Insert a day of caloric restriction into your month. Maintain your diet free of carbohydrates which now should include white sugar, white flour or rice, and the sweets from your meals. Maintain a low-carbohydrate diet. Replace the carb calories with lean meat or vegetable-based proteins.

- Reduce our carbohydrate intake.
- Replace your sweets with healthy snacks such as carrots, celery, and nut butters.
- Keep your urges for sweets satisfied with a fist-sized portion of fruit if you must.
- Couple fruit with proteins like nuts and nut butters that will help you process the fruit's natural sugar more slowly.
- Introduce yourself to a *One-Day Caloric Reduction*: and reduce your caloric intake to about 600 – 800 calories. Remember that 3500 calories equals about 1 pound of fat.

Maintain your low-carbohydrate diet. Explore a bi-weekly caloric reduction one day every two weeks. Adjust your caloric reduction schedule to one day a week or one day a month depending on your lifestyle and goals. Explore the foods that you may be sensitive to. Cut back as needed based on your reactions.

- Review the interconnection between the food you eat and the reaction you have to them.
- Identify foods that lead to an adverse reaction and consider an alternative or a replacement.

Do not forget to Live Your Life. No diet is worth living a miserable life. A happy life is a life lived in balance. Temper whatever you decide to do with the understanding that you were put here for a reason. Enjoy the life that you have. Simply do it with moderation and in a mindful way. You don't have to look like anyone else. You don't have to be someone else's idea of beauty. You simply need to be comfortable with who you are in a healthy way.

Being comfortable with who you are is the true secret to being beautiful.

Always look for the most natural, local, unprocessed foods you can find. You can always go healthier. Just start with what you know and explore your diet as you become more aware of your body and your needs. The following are foods you should look for when first start to think of your menu and your dietary habits.

Meats: if you are going to eat meat the closer your meat was raised to its natural state the better. Farms use antibiotics, hormones and reduced living conditions. Natural settings lead to natural products, and you can taste and feel the difference. If you need to eat meat look for meats such as:

- Fish and shellfish
- Duck, turkey or naturally raised poultry
- Lean pork
- Buffalo & game meats, such as rabbit & venison
- High proteins vegetables: including:
    - Kale, Spinach
    - Cruciform Vegetables such as Bok Choy, Broccoli, Brussels Sprouts, Cabbage, Cauliflower
    - Beans, Lentils, Peas
    - Squash, Zucchini, Eggplant
    - Mushrooms
    - Asparagus, Artichokes
    - Celery

- Cucumbers
- Onions
- Fruits, including:
    - Apples, Pears, Apricots,
    - Lemons, Limes, Tangerines, Oranges, Grapefruits
    - Cherries
    - Raspberries
    - Kiwis
    - Strawberries
    - Tomatoes

Life is one big beautiful adventure if you allow it to be. Spread your arms wide and laugh into all it has to offer you. You may be surprised with how happy you can be when you give yourself permission to simply embrace every experience for the joy it offers; and that goes for the people, places, work and locations you end up in and with.

I hope you have as much fun using this book as I have had in writing it. Creating a more mindful and meditative life for yourself should not be a chore, it should simply flow from who you are now to who you want to be.

Don't worry, you do not have to be happy all the time, nobody is. You do not have to make the right choice at every decision-point, nobody ever does. Just don't beat yourself up when you don't. Acknowledge your mistake and get on with your life. Mistakes are what make life fun and exciting, if you allow them to.

Sometimes it is the mistakes we make that remind us we are alive. The most memorable vacations we have are the ones where not everything goes according to plan.

The secret to living a full life is to surround yourself
with good people and to mix it up from time to
time. Invite people you may not know all that well
to your dinners, do things that take you out of your
comfort zone, take a calculated risk from time to
time and see where it leads you. Most important
laugh at whatever life throws your way. This is
what truly living is all about.

Use this book as a starting point to curate your life
in the direction you want it to go and for refining
your life into a more meditative and mindful life
that fits who you truly are. Use the mindful
practices that I have presented to you throughout
your life to slow it down, to remove the toxins and
to enjoy the Love and the positivity in all things, be
they people, news, music, work and even attitudes
you run into.

Embrace them all, because they are yours.
Be well and with Love,

Jeff

Recipes for Mindful Eating

You come from the earth. You will return to the earth when you pass. Between those two moments the earth will always heal you if you allow it to. There is tea to help you wake, there is lavender to help you sleep. When you walk in the woods you feel refreshed, when you watch the surf roll from a beach you feel calmed. Food heals in the same way that a mountain path or ocean beach does. It puts you in connection with the planet we all share, which is why the closer your food is to its natural state the greater is its ability to calm, to refresh, and to heal.

A healthy meal does more than feed your body, it nourishes your mind and spirit as well. When you share your table with friends and loved ones you will feel the love of your community and the connection you have with those who share your table.

You need to eat, so allow your mealtime to be your connection to the people and the earth around you in a calm and loving way. Your sangha starts with you. All you have to do is open your heart and share your meal with those you love. Even if your meal is just a cup of tea on a park bench the act of sharing will turn every bite into an ever-widening circle of connection to enjoy the company of others.

This is what Mindful Eating is all about. It starts with you and expands outward to the community that you are a part of, connecting you in love and health. You will lose weight along the way, but more important you will feel what it is to rise above as your mind and spirit shed the weight that has kept you shackled to the ground in the past.

The following recipes are quick and delicious meals designed for two people. Use them to replace your current repertoire of every-day meals you have come to rely on. Many come from recipes that I have cooked for years replacing standby ingredients with healthier options.

In some I replaced sugar with honey or maple syrup, in other I have replaced white potatoes with sweet potatoes, in others still I have swapped out white flour for chickpea flour to create gluten free options. I encourage you to keep this evolution going so that they become yours.

The more you cook, the more you will realize that Mindful Eating does not start at your table. It begins with the menu you plan and the ingredients you find. Take your time, create a menu for yourself, then change that menu based on what is in season and available.

Connect your body with your food. Read the ingredients and learn about what you are putting into your body. As you learn to shop you will begin to look for fresher, more locally sourced proteins that are native to your region. You learn to shop with all six of your senses, smelling the freshness, feeling the firmness, and reaching out with your heart as you connect yourself to everything you bring home.

When you shop mindfully, you will find it is no longer a task, but an opportunity to connect with your food and yourself on a whole other level. Food is about so much more than just supplying your body with the nutrients it needs. Food is the fuel that you may have been taking for granted all these years. Share you knowledge with those around you and get them excited about the new path you are all about to embark on, you will be happier for it.

Enjoy and be well.

There is a reason this recipe is the first one. It is simple, easy, vegetarian and Paleo friendly. It is also delicious, around which to build your repertoire of meals. It can be served to your family or at a formal sitting with great results. Most of the people I have shared it with quickly learn to make meatless meatballs or even burgers out of this recipe. I have been asked for this recipe so often that once you try it I doubt you will ever return to eating meat again.

Information:
Servings: 2-6
Active Time: 30 minutes, Total Time: 60 minutes

Ingredients
1-2 Tbs. extra-virgin olive oil
4 cloves garlic, (smashed)
1 medium eggplant (unpeeled, cut into 1" cubes)
1 medium onion (rough chop)
½ cup fresh Italian parsley leaves (chopped)
¼ cup fresh basil (chopped)
1 cup grated vegan parmesan
1 cup almond meal
1 egg white
Salt & pepper to taste

Directions

Preheat oven to 350 degrees.
Spread onion, garlic and eggplant on a baking sheet.
Drizzle with oil and toss lightly. Bake for 10 – 15
minutes until softened and the edges begin to
darken.

Place roasted vegetables and herbs into a food
processor and pulse until well chopped, but not
pureed. You want to have some chunks that will
add texture to your meatballs.

Transfer eggplant mixture to a large mixing bowl.
Add cheese, almond meal and egg white and stir to
combine well. This mixture can be refrigerated,
covered for up to a day.

Roll mixture into golf ball sized 1 ½ " balls and
place on a lightly oiled baking sheet.
Bake for 25 minutes, without turning until firm on
the outside and browned underneath.
Transfer meatballs to a large saucepan and cover
with our quick tomato sauce

Simmer for 10-20 minutes, or longer as your tastes
call for.

Who said falafel had to be fried? The first time I cooked this recipe I tried frying or sautéing them and found they soaked up the oil liked sponges. That was when I started baking mine. They have that same wonderful crust you get from frying with a fraction of the calories and no loss of flavor.

Information:
Servings 2-4
Active Time: 20 minutes
Total Time: 60 minutes

Ingredients
2 cups cooked chickpeas. (2 cans drained)
3 - 4 scallions, greens rough chopped
2 cloves garlic, peeled, smashed & coarsely chopped
1/4 cup chopped parsley
1/4 cup chopped cilantro
1 egg
1 lemon, juiced
1-2 teaspoons ground cumin
1-2 teaspoons ground coriander
Scant pinch cayenne pepper
Salt & Pepper to taste
1 1/2 teaspoons baking powder
1/4 - 1/2 cup chickpea flour

Directions

In a food processor - combine the chickpeas, scallions, garlic, cumin, coriander, cayenne, parsley, cilantro, egg, and lemon juice. Pulse to combine into a rough paste with visible chunks.

Season with salt and pepper. Add 1/4 cup of the chickpea flour and pulse to combine. Continue to add flour as needed until the paste resembles a wet dough. Remove to a bowl and chill in the refrigerator for 30 minutes.

Preheat your oven to 400 degrees. Lightly oil a baking sheet and remove the falafel mixture from your refrigerator. Add the baking powder and stir well to combine thoroughly. Drop large Tbs. and place them on a lightly oiled cookie sheet with about an inch or two between them.

Bake for twenty minutes and gently turn each falafel patty over. Return to the oven for another twenty minutes until golden brown and cooked through.

Serve with sliced cherry tomatoes, cucumbers, radishes and White Bean Sauce (recipe follows).

Chicken Shawarma is wonderful on its own or as an accompaniment to a plate of falafel. Treat your friends and family to a low-key, mid-week meal that is easy, filling and healthy.

Information:
Servings 2-4
Time: 30 minutes active, 2+ hours with marinating

Ingredients
2 lemons, juiced
½ cup olive oil, + 1 - 2 Tbs.
6 cloves garlic, peeled, smashed and minced
1 teaspoon kosher salt
2 teaspoons freshly ground black pepper
2 teaspoons ground cumin
2 teaspoons paprika
½ teaspoon turmeric
 A pinch ground cinnamon
 Red-pepper flakes, to taste
2 pounds boneless, skinless chicken thighs
1 large red onion, peeled and cut into eighths
2 Tbs. chopped fresh parsley

Directions - Marinade

Combine lemon juice, olive oil, garlic, salt, pepper, cumin, paprika, turmeric, cinnamon and red-pepper flakes in a bowl and stir to combine
Add the chicken, and toss well to coat. Cover and place in your refrigerator for at least 1 hour and up to 8 hours.

Directions - Cooking

Preheat your oven to 425. Grease a baking sheet with the remaining tablespoon of olive oil. Cut the red onion into eighths leaving the segments connected by the stalk base. Add the red onion to the chicken marinade and toss lightly to combine. Remove the chicken and onion from the marinade, spread evenly across the pan. Drizzle with the remaining marinade.

Place the chicken in your oven, and roast for 30-40 minutes, until it is browned and cooked through.

Remove from the oven and allow to rest for 5 minutes. Heat a sauté pan with 2 Tbs. olive oil. Crisp the chicken over high heat until it begins to brown and curl.

Serve with sliced tomatoes, radishes and white bean sauce and if you wish.

This is one of the most incredible recipes for an easy meal that receives rave reviews every time I serve it. Family and friends, vegan, vegetarian or carnivorous will all want more.

Information
Servings 2-4
Active Time: 30 minutes, Total Time 1 hour

Ingredients - Gnocchi
1-lb sweet potato
1 Tbs. olive oil
1/4 cup vegan Parmesan cheese
1/2 tsp salt
1 1/4 cup gluten-free flour (garbanzo or chick pea flour)

Ingredients - Sauce
8 tablespoons ghee
1 cloves garlic
¼ cup sage leaves (cut into thin strips)
1/4 cup almond milk
1 teaspoon sea salt
1/2 cup vegan Parmesan cheese

Directions
Peel and cut sweet potato into rough 1" chunks.
Heat olive oil in a covered sauce pot
Add sweet potatoes and brown on each side (3-5
minutes/side)
Add ¼ cup water, cover and steam for 5-10 minutes
until fork tender

Place baked sweet potatoes in a bowl and mash.
Add parmesan and salt until well combined.
Add flour, 1/2 cup at a time, and gently knead the
mixture after each addition. Be careful not to over-
knead as your gnocchi will get tough.
Transfer your dough to a clean and lightly floured
work surface.
Form it into a 9" × 5" shape.

Cut off a 1" slice to work with and roll that into a
¾" rope. As you roll, gently separate your fingers to
lengthen your rope. If your rope gets too long,
simply cut it into a more manageable length. Cut
your rope into 1-inch segments. These are your
gnocchi.

Using a fork, gently press the tines down on each
gnocchi and pull toward you to make slight
impressions along each piece. These will help your
gnocchi cook evenly and help your sauce cling to
the gnocchi.

Bring a large pot of salted water to boil, add your gnocchi.

Your gnocchi will be done when they float to the top.

Use a slotted spoon, transfer your cooked gnocchi to a plate and place a piece of butcher's paper between each layer or lightly drizzle with olive oil to prevent them from sticking together. Continue doing this with the remaining gnocchi.

Heat 1 Tbs of olive oil in a skillet over medium heat. Add the gnocchi and sauté until lightly browned. Place cooked gnocchi on a separate plate.

Heat ghee in a skillet over medium heat. When your ghee begins to foam add the garlic and sage, allow it to settle before adding gnocchi.

Sauté until lightly covered then add the almond milk and vegan Parmesan.

Toss gently to evenly coat the gnocchi, add a pinch of salt and pepper to taste.

Serve immediately.

Most of the vegetables can be high quality frozen vegetables, since they will boil down in this recipe. It will make it easier to keep ingredients at hand to make this delicious soup at any time.

Information
Servings 4 — 8
Total Time: 55 minutes, Active Time: 35 minutes

Ingredients
1-2 Tbsp olive oil
4 cloves garlic (minced)
1 large onion (rough dice)
4 large carrots (sliced / rough chop)
6 stalks celery (sliced / rough chop)
1 green bell pepper (rough chop)
8 oz green beans (rough chop)
16 oz chopped tomatoes (I prefer Pomi)
1/2 head cabbage (chopped into 1" cubes)
Small bunch fresh parsley, chopped
1/2 Tbsp smoked paprika
1 tsp dried oregano
1/2 tsp dried thyme
4 - 6 cups broth
1-2 Tbsp lemon juice
Salt and pepper to taste

Directions

Drizzle olive oil into sauce pan. Add the garlic and onion. Sauté over medium heat until the onions are soft and transparent.

Add the carrots, celery, bell pepper, and green beans to the pot. Add the chopped tomatoes and stir to combine.

Allow the vegetables to simmer and soften before adding the cabbage. Add the chopped parsley, paprika, oregano, thyme, and some freshly cracked pepper. Stir to combine. Add the broth (vegetable or chicken is fine)

Place a lid on the pot and bring it up to a boil. Turn the heat down to medium-low and allow to simmer until the cabbage is tender (20 minutes).

Salt and pepper to taste. Your stock may have added salt, but do not scrimp on the salt; that will add a lot of the flavor this soup calls for.

This fall soup combines only ten ingredients. It combines carrots with butternut squash and roasted acorn squash to create bowls of goodness. You can really use any type of squash for this, even sweet potatoes. It is a healthy comfort food for you to spoon into during the cold months.

Information
Servings: 4-6
Active time: 1 hour
Total time: 1 hour 30 mins

Ingredients
2 acorn squash (halved)
1 medium sized butternut squash (halved)
1 Tbsp. melted ghee or coconut butter
2 Tbsp. maple syrup
1 1/2 Tbsp. olive oil
1/2 small onion (diced)
3 cloves garlic (minced)
4 cups combined sweet potato, carrots, or butternut squash (cubed)
4 cups vegetable broth
1 tsp thyme
1 bay leaves

Preheat oven to 350 degrees
Split the squash in half

Scoop out the seeds, lightly salt and pepper to taste,
Drizzle with olive oil and maple syrup.

Place squash on a baking sheet and bake for 60 – 90
minutes, or until squash is fork tender and golden
brown on the edges (baking time depends on size).
While the squash roasts heat your oil in a large
sauce pot over medium heat.

Add onion, and garlic. Sauté for 4 minutes, until
onion is soft and transparent.

Add squash and carrots, season with salt and black
pepper and sauté for 4-5 minutes until vegetables
are slightly softened.

Add broth and herbs. Bring to a low boil over
medium-high heat. Reduce heat and simmer
uncovered for 20-30 minutes.

Use an immersion blender and puree smooth and
creamy.

When time is short, this is a quick and easy dinner for two. The roasted sweet potatoes and onions add a soulful taste to the chickpeas and dark greens. Top with an easy tahini-honey sauce and serve.

Information
Servings: 2
Active Time: 30 minutes
Total Time: 30 minutes

Ingredients - Bowl
2 Tbs. olive oil
1 small red onion, cut into wedges
1 large sweet potato, quartered lengthwise
1 small bundle broccoli rabe (larger stems removed and rough chopped)
1 large handfuls kale (stripped and rough chopped)
salt and pepper (to taste)

Ingredients - Chickpeas
2 cups chickpeas, drained rinsed + patted dry
1 clove garlic (minced)
1 tsp cumin
1/2 tsp smoked paprika (hot or mild)
1/4 tsp turmeric
Salt & pepper to taste

1/4 cup tahini
1 Tbs. honey
1/2 lemon (juiced)
3-4 Tbs. hot water to thin

Directions
Preheat oven to 350 degrees.

Whip tahini with a fork add lemon juice, honey and hot water to create a pourable sauce.

Drizzle olive oil into a skillet and heat over medium-high. Stir in spices and chickpeas, sauté to ensure chickpeas are evenly covered and browned. Remove from heat and set aside.

Lightly oil a baking sheet. Add sweet potatoes, skin-side down, and onion wedges drizzle lightly with olive oil, and bake for 20 min.

Turn sweet potatoes and add broccoli. Bake for another 15 minutes. Place kale on top of roasted vegetables, drizzle with olive oil, season with salt and pepper and bake for another 5 minutes.

Arrange kale and broccoli on a plate. Arrange sweet potatoes and onions on top of the kale, add chickpeas and drizzle with tahini sauce.

Everyone has a vegan take on the classic Sheppard's Pie these days. This one was adapted from my mother who tended to make it with the left-overs at the end of the week. I think that's probably the way it was meant to be made, but I refined it with the usual alterations to make it as healthy as possible, replacing the white potato topping with a sweet potatoes and ground beef for bison or turkey.

Information
Servings: 6-8
Active Time: 20 – 30 min., Total Time: 30 – 60 min.

Ingredients
Filling
1 lb. ground grass-fed bison or ground turkey
3 medium carrots, (diced)
½ green pepper (diced)
½ cup peas (frozen are fine)
1 small onion (diced)
2 cloves garlic (minced)
½ tsp. rosemary
1 tsp. smoked paprika
6 Tbs. tomato paste
1 Tbs. almond meal
salt & pepper (to taste)

Topping
2 medium sweet potatoes (cut into rough 1" cubes)
1 Tbsp. olive oil
½ tsp cayenne
salt & pepper to taste

Directions
Preheat oven to 350°F.

Combine the almond meal and water and set aside.
Sauté the bison or turkey In a skillet on medium
heat until lightly browned.

Add the chopped vegetables and cook over medium
heat until soft (about 10 minutes). Once soft, stir in
tomato paste, almond mixture, and season with salt
and pepper.

Make the topping while the filling cooks, add 1 Tbs.
olive oil to a sauce pot and add sweet potatoes. Stir
to brown on all sides. Add ¼ cup of water, cover,
and steam until fork tender (about 5 minutes). Mash
well.

Transfer the meat filling to a 9" casserole dish, top
with the Sweet Potatoes, bake for 15 minutes and
serve.

This delicious Orange Chicken recipe replaces the sugar with honey and uses fresh orange juice and zest to provide the bright flavors with a sprinkle of red pepper flakes to add a kick.

Information
Servings: 4 - 6
Active Time: 20 minutes, Total Time 45 minutes

Ingredients
1 lb chicken thighs (skinless & boneless)
2 Tbs. arrow root
¼ cup cold water
2 Tbs. soy sauce
1 clove garlic (minced)
1 teaspoon ginger (grated)
2 large oranges (zested & juiced)
2 1/2 teaspoons of sambal chili sauce
2 Tbs. mirin
3 Tbs. white/rice wine vinegar
3 Tbs. honey
¼ teas red pepper flakes
4 green onions
1/4 teaspoon pepper
1 teaspoon salt

Directions – Orange Sauce

In a small bowl, make an arrowroot slurry by combining ¼ cup water and 2 Tbs. arrowroot. Set aside.

Remove zest and juice your oranges to produce approximately 2 Tbs. of zest and 1 cup of fresh juice.

In a small saucepan reduce the orange juice to ¾ cup over a low simmer.
Add the zest, soy sauce, garlic, ginger, chili sauce, mirin, rice wine/white wine vinegar, honey, red pepper flakes, pepper and salt to taste.
Increase heat to medium, stirring occasionally.

Whisk in the arrow root slurry and continue to cook until the sauce begins to thicken, about 2 minutes.

Remove from heat and set aside.

Directions – Chicken

Cut chicken thighs into bite-sized pieces. Add chicken to a bowl and dust with 1 Tbs. arrowroot and shake to coat. (Do not worry about fully coating each piece, just a dusting is fine.)

Heat 2 Tbs. olive oil and sauté the chicken pieces over medium high heat, until the chicken is lightly browned, firm and crisp.

Add the orange sauce to the chicken and cook until
the sauce starts to bubble and all pieces are coated,
about 1 to 5 minutes.

Sprinkle with green onions and serve immediately.

Tired of having vegetarian burgers that try to taste like meat but just fail to hit the mark? This recipe takes a different turn. They are delicious on their own with the dark tastes of black beans perfectly balanced with the rich taste of walnuts.

Information
Servings: 4
Time: 30 Minutes

Ingredients
1 cup cooked brown rice (recipe follows)
1 cup walnuts (raw)
1 tsp olive oil
1/2 onion (diced)
1/4 tsp chili powder
1 tsp cumin
1/2 tsp smoked paprika
1/2 tsp each sea salt and black pepper
1 Tbs. cane sugar
1 1/2 cups black beans (cooked)
1/3 cup almond meal
3-4 Tbs. vegan BBQ sauce (I prefer Wild Thymes Thai One on BBQ Sauce)

Directions

Bring 2 cups of water to a boil. Add 1 cup of brown rice. Reduce heat to low and cover with a tight-fitting lid for 20 - 30 minutes. Uncover and fluff with a fork.

Brown walnuts over medium heat. Shake pan and stir frequently for 5 - 7 minutes or until fragrant and lightly browned. Remove from pan and set aside to cool.

Sauté onion in olive oil until soft and translucent. Season with salt and pepper, remove from heat, and set aside.

Process walnuts, chili powder, cumin, smoked paprika, salt, pepper and cane sugar in a blender. Pulse until it resembles a fine meal. Set aside. Mash black beans until only a few whole beans are left.

Combine cooked rice, walnut mixture, onion, and BBQ sauce. Mix thoroughly until a moldable dough forms. If dry add additional 1-2 Tbs.p BBQ sauce. Divide into patties and cook in a sauté pan. Sear over medium-high heat on one side. Once browned gently turn, cover and cook for 3-4 minutes more.

This is one of the easiest mid-week dinners I know. Dress it up with a batch of baked sweet potato fries and a kale salad, or dive into them on their own. This is perfect for a quick stove-top meal in a skillet with a lid to help keep the juices in. Secret - I use a small bit of water to finish the burgers off by steaming them and create a bit of au jus on the side.

Information
Servings 4
Time: 30 minutes total, 10 minutes active

Ingredients
1 lbs. ground turkey
4 – 8 romaine lettuce leaves
1 Tbs. olive oil
1/8 tsp red pepper flakes
Salt & pepper to taste
1/4 cup water (scant)

Directions
Form the turkey into patties and salt and pepper generously. Allow to rest and firm up in the refrigerator for half an hour.

Heat the olive oil in a pan over medium high heat. Rotate the pan to coat evenly. When it begins to glisten, add the turkey patties and sear.

Lower the heat to medium. Allow to cook, without nudging, lifting, or otherwise moving them. Let them form a nice sear to prevent them from drying out or sticking when it is time to flip. Cook for 7 - 10 minutes or until the meat has turned white for about 1/4 inch from the bottom.

Turn and cover. Continue to cook for another 5-7 minutes before adding a small amount of water. Allow them to steam for a few minutes.

Remove the lid and continue to cook, shaking the pan until the water darkens and reduces into a brothy au jus.

Wrap in the romaine leaves and serve with a kale salad and baked sweet potato fries.

This is a healthy alternative to the traditional egg-based breakfast burrito. Tofu works extremely well when squeezed of all water and cooked quickly.

Information
Servings: 2 - 4
Time: 20 Minutes

Ingredients
1 medium sized head of cauliflower
1 Lb. tofu (extra firm)
1 Tbs. olive oil
1 clove garlic
½ onion (diced)
1 medium bell pepper (diced)
½ teaspoon thyme
½ teaspoon oregano
1/4 teaspoon turmeric
½ teaspoon smoked paprika

Directions
Remove stems from cauliflower and cut florets into small segments. Pulse in a food processor until they resemble a coarse couscous.

Sauté garlic and onion in a heavy gauge skillet until
translucent. Add bell pepper and cauliflower. Cook
until just starting to brown - about 3 - 5 minutes.
Add the herbs and seasoning.

Break tofu apart with your fingers. Add to your pan
and stir as you would any scramble.
Remove from heat and wrap in a tortilla with your
choice of salsa for a light and nutritious breakfast
burrito.

This white bean sauce is a wonderful accompaniment to our baked Falafel or our Chicken Shawarma. It is also wonderful on its own as a dip for vegetables.

The yogurt is optional. It adds a nice creaminess to the sauce, but an alternative is slowly adding water to the sauce to make it creamier.

Information
Servings 2-4
Time: 20 minutes active, 20 minutes total

Ingredients
3/4 cup cooked white beans (cannellini)
1 small clove garlic, peeled, smashed & coarsely chopped
1/2 lemon, juiced
2 Tbs. olive oil
Kosher salt and freshly ground black pepper
1/4 cup Greek yogurt

Directions
Combine all ingredients in a food processor and pulse to combine.

Depending on the consistency desired, add cold water 1 tablespoon at a time after yogurt is added.

As its name implies, this is a quick and easy tomato sauce. It is not a refined Italian tomato sauce that a finer chef would produce, but a sauce meant for real people with real schedules that is clean, healthy and delicious.

Information
Servings: 6 – 8
Active Time: 20 minutes, Total Time: 40 minutes

Ingredients
1 Tbs. olive oil
1 clove garlic
1 small onion
1/8 tsp basil (direct or fresh)
1 tsp tomato paste
½ tsp anchovy paste
8 oz. chopped tomatoes (I prefer Pomi off season)
Pinch salt & pepper (to taste)
Pinch red pepper flakes (Optional)

Directions
Heat olive oil over medium high heat. Sauté the garlic and onion until softened and just translucent.

Add the basil, anchovy and tomato paste. Give a
quick stir and add the chopped tomatoes and
reduce the heat to a low simmer for 10 – 20 minutes.
Add salt, pepper and pepper flakes to taste.

Add vegetable noodles or eggplant meatballs and
saute, or pour over your favorite pasta for a
satisfying meal.

This classic dip is a mainstay in our house. We have been known to make a batch for the week and watch it disappear as dinner on that first night. Enjoy it any way you wish.

Information
Servings: 4-6 as a dip
Time: 10 Minutes

Ingredients
One 15-ounce can chickpeas or garbanzo beans
1 large lemon juiced
1/4 cup Tahini or sesame seed paste
1 garlic clove, peels, smashed and minced
2 Tbs. olive oil, + drizzle for serving
Sale & Pepper to taste
1/2 tsp ground cumin
2 to 3 Tbs. water

Directions
Combine all ingredients except water in a food processor and pulse until smooth. Add water 1 Tbs. at a time until the desired consistency is reached. Place in a bowl, refrigerate until ready to serve.

Serve with slivered carrots, celery, squash, zucchini, radishes, or cherry tomatoes.

Information
Servings 2-4
Active Time - 15 - 20 Minutes, Total Time: 15 – 29
Minutes

Ingredients
1 Head Cauliflower

Directions
Do not cook the cauliflower ahead of time.
Remove florets from stalk.

Add several cauliflower florets to a food processor a
little at a time.

Pulse until it takes on the consistency and texture of
couscous or rice.

Set aside for cooking, or place in freezer. At this
stage your cauliflower rice / couscous will keep in
the freezer for several months.

Who said fries need to be fried in a vat of heart-clogging oil? You will find Baked Sweet Potato Fries are a great, high fiber, addition that go well with almost any meal. They are a healthy alternative that taste great. Better still, even a small sweet potato will give you more fries than two people can eat. Well, almost…

Information
Servings: 2-4
Active Time: 10 Minutes, Total Time: 60 Minutes

Ingredients
1 or 2 Sweet Potatoes
2 Tbs. Olive Oil
Salt & Pepper to taste

Directions
Preheat oven to 375 degrees.
Slice the sweet potato into 1/2" - 3/4" slices and arrange on a baking sheet. Drizzle with olive oil and lightly toss as you salt & pepper to taste. Bake for 20 - 30 minutes until browned on the bottom.
Remove from the oven and gently turn.
Bake for another 15 - 20 minutes until browned on all sides. Be careful not to burn, as they will blacken quickly.

I know, but seriously, who can resist a batch of fresh kale chips at any time, day or night. It's a great alternative to processed chips, and they are easier to make that my may think.

Information
Servings: 2-4
Active Time: 10 Minutes
Total Time: 40 Minutes

Ingredients
8 oz. Kale (Tuscan or San San Lacinato)
2 Tbs. Olive Oil
Salt & Pepper to taste

Directions

Preheat oven to 350 degrees.
Shred the kale leaves by tearing away from stalk and pulling stalk through the thumb and fore-finger of your hand. Chop or rear the leaves into large, rough chip-sized portions.

Lightly toss the soon-to-be chips in olive, until complete coated. Arrange on a baking sheet in a single layer as you salt & pepper to taste.

Bake for 20 - 40 minutes until crisp and crunchy. It will depend on the water content of the kale.

Remove from the oven and enjoy.

This simple and salad brings a wonderful tahini dressing together with a slaw-like crunch of shredded brussels sprouts and toasted almonds. The miso lends a savory umami flavor for a twist on the usual.

Information
Servings: 4-6
Active Time: 20 minutes, Total Time: 40 minutes

Ingredients
1 bunch of dark greens such as kale
2 dozen small brussels sprouts
4 Tbs. slivered almonds

Directions
Using a sharp knife or the slot on a grater, shred the brussels sprouts across the grain to produce fine shreds.

Toss with the kale and drizzle with the tahini dressing that follows.

¼ cup tahini
2 Tbs. champagne vinegar
2 tsp white miso
juice of 1 lemon
pinch of red pepper flakes
¼ cup water

Directions
Remove the stalks from the kale and chop the kale leaves into small, bite-sized pieces.

Sprinkle a dash of sea salt over the kale and massage a light dribble of olive oil into the kale with your hands. Scrunch the kale gently to soften it until it becomes darker in color and fragrant.

Transfer to a serving bowl.

Trim your Brussels sprouts and slice as thin as possible. Add the sprouts to the kale, breaking up any clumps with your fingers.

In a small mixing bowl, whisk together the tahini, vinegar, miso, maple syrup and red pepper flakes. Add the water until your mixture is smooth and creamy. Pour the dressing over the kale and sprouts, mix well, and allow to rest.

In a small pan toast the almond slivers over medium heat. Stir frequently, until fragrant and golden (about five minutes).

Toss the toasted almonds with the greens and serve immediately.

For those with a bit more time, or simply wanting something more, this is a fancier salad with crunch and flavor bursts throughout. Enjoy in the Summer, Fall, Winter or Spring to set your lunch or dinner off right.

Information
Servings: 2-4
Time: 10 Minutes

Ingredients
8-12 Ounces fresh Kale (preferably Lacinato)
1/4 - 1/2 cup dried cherries or cranberries
1 Medium Apple (Pink Lady, Fuji, or similar apple with crunch) - diced
1/4 Cup Almond slivers
1/2 Lemon juiced

Dressing
1 Small clove garlic, peeled, smashed and minced
1/4 Teas salt
3 Tbs. Olive oil
1 Tbs. Champagne vinegar
3 Tbs. Dijon-style mustard
Salt & Pepper to taste

Strip the leaves from the stalk by tearing the base of the leaves free and stripping the leaves through the thumb and forefinger of one hand.

Chop into large rough segments. Combine in a large bowl with dried fruit, diced apples and almond slivers. Drizzle with lemon juice to prevent apples from discoloring.

For the dressing, place minced garlic in bottom of a small bowl or glass. Add the 1/2 teaspoon salt and allow the salt to absorb the garlic's flavor, about 15 minutes.

Before serving, add olive oil, Dijon-style mustard, champagne vinegar and pepper to taste. Stir to combine thoroughly and give the dressing enough time to flavor the kale before serving.

For anyone who just wants a quick and easy salad at any time. You cannot get any easier than this. Tear, oil, sprinkle with salt and pepper, and voila! enjoy on its own or with another main dish. the lemon is a nice addition, but if you are in a hurry, simple olive oil will do.

Information
Servings: 2-4 Time: 10 Minutes

Ingredients
8-12 Ounces fresh Kale (preferably Tuscan or Lacinato)
1 medium lemon juiced
Salt & Pepper to taste
1/4 Cup Olive Oil - to taste
Parmesan Cheese (Optional & to taste)

Directions
Strip the leaves from the stalk by pulling the stems through your thumb and forefinger, stripping the leaves. Chop into large rough segments.

Drizzle with olive oil and lemon juice, salt and pepper, parmesan cheese, and toss to combine. Allow to marinate before serving.

Information
Servings: 1 Quart
Active Time: 10 Minutes, Total Time: 8 Hours

Ingredients
1 cup raw almonds
4 cups filtered water

Directions:
Soak the almonds in filtered water overnight or for
8 – 24 hours.

Strain out water and add almonds to a blender (I
prefer the Vitamix).

Add enough filtered water to make 4 cups.
Puree on high for about a minute.
Strain through a nut bag to remove as much almond
meal from your milk as possible.

Pour into a container and use as you wish.
Refrigerates for two weeks or more.

Reserve almond meal for use in other recipes such
as A Monk's Crackers or Eggplant Meatballs.

Almond Milk Yogurt

This is an easy recipe that I prepare every week for daily use.

Information
Servings: 1 Quart
Active Time: 10 minutes, Total Time: 8 – 12 hours

Ingredients
2 cups raw almonds (unroasted, unsalted)
2 Tbs. cane sugar
1 teaspoon agar agar powder (do not use flakes)
1/4 cup arrowroot powder
1 Qt. Filtered water
Vegan yogurt starter - I recommend culturesforhealth.com

Directions:
Sterilize all utensils, bowls and your fermentation container by filling with or dousing in boiling water.

Soak almonds in filtered water to cover 18 - 48 hours. Rinse well and drain.

Transfer almonds to a high-powered blender (vitamix is a great choice). Add enough filtered water to bring contents to the 4 cup mark.

Blend on high speed until smooth. Place a large colander over a bowl and drape with a nut-milk bag or straining cloth. Pour nut milk through bag and squeeze out as much of the milk as possible. Set almond pulp aside to use in the *A Monk's Almond Meal Crackers* or *the Eggplant Meatballs* recipes.

Pour the Almond Milk into a 2-quart measuring cup. Add enough filtered water to measure 4 cups. Pour into a pot and heat over medium-low heat. Add the Cane Sugar (do not worry, it will be digested by the bacteria in the fermentation process) to the milk and bring to 180 degrees.

Add the arrowroot to 1/2 cup of cold filtered water. Stir your arrowroot slurry into your milk mixture to combine completely. Be careful of making your arrowroot slurry too far in advance as it will clump. Remove from heat and stir until everything is incorporated.

As the milk heats, add 2 cups of filtered water to a second pot and bring to a simmer. Once simmering sprinkle the agar agar powder over the surface. Continue to simmer and whisk until the agar agar is completely dissolved (5 - 8 minutes).

Stir the agar agar into your almond milk mixture scraping as much as possible from the smaller pan. Whisk to incorporate fully. Add your arrow root slurry and combine.

Move your thermometer to your yogurt container to chill and place your yogurt container into your refrigerator and allow to cool undisturbed.

Once your milk mixture has cooled to 100-105°F, mix your yogurt starter into a small amount of the cooled yogurt before adding this to the rest of your yogurt mixture. It will help your culture adjust to the temperature.

Gently stir to incorporate thoroughly. Transfer your milk mixture to your yogurt maker. Leave undisturbed to incubate 8-12 hours.

**Note: if the yogurt is not thick enough for your taste, increase agar agar to 1 1/2 teaspoons on your next try.

**Note: if you prefer a tangier taste, incubate for 12 – 18 hours.

People usually ask about what to do with the leftover pulp after making Almond Yogurt. These crackers are the best we have found. If you have not made yogurt, you can find Almond Meal and Flax Meal anywhere that sells Bob's Red Mill Natural Foods.

Information
Servings: 36 - 48 Crackers
Time: 30 Minutes

Ingredients:
3 cups Almond Meal
1/4 cup Flax Meal
1 cup Almond Flour
1 Tbs. Salt
3 Tbs. Olive Oil
4 Tbs. Filtered Water
Pepper to taste

Directions:
Preheat your oven to 300F.

Combine dry ingredients into a large bowl and stir. Add olive oil and mix.

Depending on how moist your Almond Meal is add 3-4 Tbs. of water to form a damp dough that just holds together without being too wet.

Place half of the dough on a sheet of parchment paper. Place a second sheet of parchment paper on top of the dough and use an even rolling pin to roll out to an even thickness of 1/32" - 1/16".

Even up your dough to form a rectangle by cutting away the rough edges (a pizza cutter works great for this). Cut the dough into whatever sized crackers you want (1" x 2" is perfect for hummus). Slide the parchment paper and dough onto a cookie sheet.

Bake for 15 minutes. Remove cookie sheet and rotate for evenness. Continue baking for another 15 - 20 minutes or until dry and lightly browned on the edges. Remove from oven and gently lift and break apart the crackers with a spatula or knife.

Turn oven temperature down to 200 and continue to bake for another 20 minutes to crisp crackers.

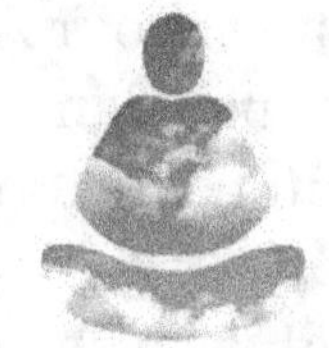

Simple Truth LLC
1 Little West 12th Street, New York NY 10014
info@simple-truth.com

i http://www.webmd.com/diet/features/lose-weight-eat-breakfast
ii http://www.drweil.com/drw/u/QAA401300/Does-Intermittent-Fasting-Promote-Weight-Loss.html
iii http://www.eurekalert.org/pub_releases/2011-04/imc-sfr033111.php
iv http://www.cmaj.ca/content/early/2013/04/08/cmaj.109-4451.full.pdf
v An excellent source of information about caloric restriction can be found through Dr. Michael Mosley.
Vihttp://www.merckmanuals.com/home/childrens_health_issues/hereditary_metabolic_disorders/disorders_of_carbohydrate_metabolism.html vii http://www.globalhealingcenter.com/sugar-problem/refined-sugar-the-sweetest-poison-of-all
viii Laurentine ten Bosch, Producer - 'Food Matters'http://foodmatters.tv/articles-1/top-10-food-additives-to-avoid